Unlock Your Home Workout Potential

Build Your Dream Physique

Peter Shark

COPYRIGHT

Unlocking Your Home Workout Potential: A Guide to Building Your Dream Physique

COPYRIGHT © 2023 BY Peter Shark

All rights reserved

CONTENTS

INTRODUCTION

Whenever you aren't ready to embark on a fitness journey, it's easy to find a thousand reasons why you shouldn't start. Yet, when that moment of readiness strikes, just one compelling reason can set you on a path to accomplishing your fitness goals.

Deep down, many of us harbor the desire for a physique that fills us with pride, one that reflects our hard work and dedication. We yearn for those moments when we gaze into the mirror, our smiles reflecting the admiration we have for our body's transformation.

If this desire for fitness is universal, then why do so many people hesitate to commit to an exercise routine that could help them achieve it? There are several factors contributing to this reluctance, with a prevalent misconception being that effective fitness can only be achieved through gym visits or hiring personal trainers. However, this couldn't be further from the truth.

You can achieve an effective workout plan that enhances your muscles and physique right in the comfort of your own home. The key ingredients? Access to the right information, unwavering dedication, and steadfast commitment.

This comprehensive guide is designed to provide you with the knowledge you need. Inside, you'll discover valuable information on how to create your home workout plan and receive essential tips to help you stay the course.

By the end of your journey, you'll not only appreciate the physical benefits but also the profound mental health advantages that accompany these home-based fitness activities.

Understanding Home Workouts

In the realm of fitness, we often hear about the benefits of gym memberships and personal trainers. These experts possess a wealth of knowledge and experience, capable of tailoring fitness routines that yield impressive results.

It's undeniable that their guidance can be invaluable. However, it's essential to recognize that building muscle, shedding excess weight, and achieving your fitness goals don't always require the traditional gym setting or the services of a personal trainer.

If you've been paying attention to the fitness landscape, you may have noticed a significant trend: the proliferation of home workout enthusiasts. True, the internet is awash with fitness content, and not everything you encounter online is reliable. Some individuals may post misleading information purely for likes and compliments.

But beneath the social media noise, a growing number of people are genuinely transforming their physical appearances without ever setting foot in a gym. The secret lies in their dedication and commitment to a home workout plan.

Defining a Home Workout Plan

A home workout plan is a thoughtfully designed and structured fitness routine aimed at enhancing your physical appearance through a series of exercises. While specialized equipment and facilities can certainly enhance the process, they are by no means mandatory.

You don't have to empty your wallet to break a sweat, shed those extra pounds, or sculpt your muscles. With the right plan and exercises, you can embark on your fitness journey with minimal or no financial investment.

Key Elements of a Home Workout Plan

Just like any activity, there are vital components that are integral to the success of your home workout plan. Once these features are missing, you'll only have a plan but will never execute it. They include:

Purpose

When you fail to define the reason for an activity, it will eventually become redundant. You need to ask yourself why you need to start regular exercise. Do you want to start so that you can post a picture on your social media profile? Do you want to do it because it is the current trend? If your reason is flimsy, you'll stop very soon.

Therefore, you have to ensure that you have a clearly defined objective before starting your plan. Endeavor to write your targets down so that you can tailor your plans in the right direction. Your goals will also help you to develop an effective diet plan that will support your commitment to physical activity.

Vision

A vision is something you see long before it happens. Having a clear vision about the kind of person you want to be determines the kind of commitment you'll have today. It enables you to channel your energy and resources in the right direction.

The purpose of starting a workout will affect your vision. Meanwhile, your vision will determine the kind of exercises you'll perform. For example, if you're doing exercise to develop your abs, you'll not have a workout plan that encourages the development of butt muscles. The kind of physique you imagine yourself having is what will determine your routine.

Gradual Process

Nothing you do in a hurry can stand the test of time. Rushing may earn you some quick results, but you'll not be able to sustain it. Besides, impatience often leads to desperation, which often leads to disastrous outcomes. In the context of physical activities, it can make you engage in strenuous routines that can have adverse effects on your health.

You must never forget that developing your physique is a gradual process. Impatience and desperation can make you injure yourself or become discouraged along the way. You need to enjoy the process to make your home workout plan a success. It is good to use the body shape of others as inspiration, but you must never forget that it took them time to achieve that physique.

Motivation

The fuel of any aspiration is passion. Zeal spurs you to follow up on a plan or strategy to ensure that you succeed. Your home workout plan will never become a reality when you lack motivation. You must be excited to do your press-ups every day.

Once you lose the desire to go on, you'll quit. So, use your vision as a springboard to get going, especially during days when you're tired or in a bad mood. Joining a fitness club may encourage you to sustain your momentum. Nonetheless, if you're self-motivated, you can still be consistent all by yourself.

Commitment

You cannot separate motivation and commitment. When you're motivated to carry out a task, you'll commit to it. A plan that lacks commitment will only remain on paper but will never be executed. Laziness is one of those factors that can stop you from achieving your desired body shape.

So, ensure that you don't allow laxity and boredom to set in. Anyone can start working out, but only committed people can sustain the momentum in the long run.

Exercise Selection

A well-crafted plan includes a variety of exercises that target different muscle groups, ensuring a balanced and comprehensive approach to fitness.

Routine Structure

A structured routine outlines when and how often you'll perform your workouts, ensuring consistency and progress tracking.

Goal Alignment

Your plan should align with your fitness goals, whether it's weight loss, muscle gain, or improved overall health.

Adaptability

An effective plan can evolve as your fitness level progresses, preventing plateaus and monotony.

Minimal Investment, Maximum Gains

One of the remarkable aspects of a home workout plan is its accessibility to virtually anyone. You can embark on your fitness journey with minimal financial investment while reaping substantial rewards for your dedication and hard work. It's about understanding that you have the power to transform your physique right from the comfort of your own home, and you can do it on your terms.

In the chapters that follow, we'll delve deeper into the components of a successful home workout plan, helping you design a routine that aligns with your goals and lifestyle.

Whether you're a beginner or a seasoned fitness enthusiast, the principles we'll explore will guide you toward achieving the results you desire without the need for an expensive gym membership or a personal trainer.

The Interplay between Physical Health and Mental Health

The intricate connection between physical health and mental well-being is undeniable; they are intertwined in ways that significantly impact our overall health. Understanding this interplay is crucial as it sheds light on the importance of maintaining both aspects for a truly holistic state of wellness.

The Holistic Definition of Health

According to the World Health Organization, health is a comprehensive concept that encompasses both physical and psychological well-being. To be truly "healthy," an individual's physical and mental health must be in harmony.

Additionally, social well-being plays a pivotal role in this holistic definition of health, further underlining the interconnectedness of these facets.

Chronic Diseases and Mental Health

Poor physical health can cast a shadow on your mental well-being. When battling a chronic disease, the emotional toll can be immense. Conditions like diabetes, for instance, can lead to feelings of depression due to the constant management and lifestyle adjustments required.

Experts have observed that individuals with schizophrenia face a doubled risk of dying from heart disease and a tripling of the risk of respiratory disease-related fatalities. This heightened risk can be attributed to the lack of routine health checks for mental health patients, which neglect crucial parameters like weight, blood pressure, and cholesterol.

Depression and Its Effects on Lifestyle

Depression and anxiety can take a toll on your eating habits and exercise routines. When struggling with mental health issues, it's common to find yourself either overindulging in unhealthy foods or neglecting nutrition altogether.

The motivation to exercise may wane, leading to a sedentary lifestyle that adversely affects physical health. Research findings highlight that individuals with low self-esteem are 32% more likely to succumb to cancer, and depression increases the risk of coronary heart disease. This connection stems from the profound influence of mental health on dietary choices and adherence to a healthy lifestyle.

Scientific research has solidified the link between regular exercise and mental health. Physical activity influences the release and uptake of endorphins, the brain's "feel-good" chemicals. Consequently, a lack of exercise increases susceptibility to depression, emphasizing the importance of physical activity in maintaining mental well-being.

The positive impact of physical exercise extends to mental alertness. Studies have shown that engaging in physical activities can generate positive energy and sharpen cognitive functions. Even short bursts of exercise, such as a brisk ten-minute walk, can make a significant difference in enhancing mental alertness and overall cognitive vitality.

Understanding the intricate interplay between physical health and mental well-being underscores the necessity of nurturing both aspects of health for a fulfilling and healthy life. By recognizing these connections, you empower yourself to make informed choices that promote holistic well-being.

CHAPTER 2: THE MOTIVATION BEHIND HOME WORKOUTS

In today's interconnected world, the rise of social media has brought us closer to countless influences from around the globe. While this can be a source of inspiration, it can also lead to a desire to conform and fit in with the crowd, fearing rejection or judgment.

This inclination to follow trends and appease others can even extend to your home workout plan. You might find yourself wanting to embark on a fitness journey to meet the standards set by people who may not genuinely care about your well-being.

The last thing you want is people paying attention to you unnecessarily because of your physique. Unfortunately, this is the experience of many people today, especially plus-size individuals.

The internet and media are rife with insensitive jokes that mock people for their weight. While excessive weight may not be beneficial for your appearance and can pose health risks, you should approach your workout plan with the right mindset.

Acceptance and Self-Love

Before diving into your workout plan, it's crucial to accept and love yourself as you are. Your fitness journey should not be fueled by a desire to avoid unwarranted attention or negative comments. Remember, the transformation of your body is a gradual process. You should certainly have a vision of your desired physique, but it's equally important to value yourself as you are now.

Choosing Supportive Friends

Surround yourself with friends who support and respect you, regardless of your appearance. If your current circle often makes insensitive comments about your looks, it might be time to distance yourself from them. Good friends will acknowledge your areas for improvement and offer guidance without judgment. They will provide moral support to help you maintain your motivation.

Motivation for the Right Reasons

Some fitness advice suggests using negative comments and experiences as motivation. For example, trying to look attractive to get back at an ex-partner may seem tempting, but it stems from insecurity.

Remember, anyone who leaves you solely because of your physique doesn't deserve your time. You should never start a workout plan out of a desire for revenge.

Staying Clear of Media Pressure

Media influences can affect your self-perception more than you realize. Posting heavily edited pictures to garner likes and positive comments can lead to a false sense of self-worth. Before starting your fitness journey, examine your motives.

If you're doing it solely for social media approval or to prove a point to detractors, it's important to reconsider.

Signs You're Working out for the Wrong Reasons

Recognizing the signs of a misguided motive is crucial to maintaining a healthy fitness journey. Here are some symptoms that indicate you may be working out for the wrong reasons:

Excessive Intensity

Pushing yourself too hard due to impatience can lead to injuries.

Overly Focused

Fixating on a particular type of exercise or one side of your body instead of holistic health.

Prolonged Pain

Suffering from excessive soreness or lingering pain for a week or more.

One-Sided Discomfort

Feeling pain on one side of your body instead of evenly distributed discomfort.

These signs often manifest when you're driven by external pressures or the need to prove yourself. It's essential to realign your motives with your overall health and well-being to ensure a successful and sustainable fitness journey.

CHAPTER 3: BENEFITS OF STAYING FIT

Understanding the benefits of staying fit provides the motivation needed to maintain your workout routine. A home workout plan offers you a multitude of advantages that extend beyond mere physical appearance.

Prevents Muscle Loss

As you age, your body undergoes natural changes, and maintaining muscle mass becomes increasingly challenging. Muscles that you've worked hard to build can degrade over time, leading to a less attractive and functional physique. However, you can proactively address this issue through regular exercise.

Investing in a consistent workout regimen can help you not only maintain but also increase your muscle mass, regardless of your age. It's not uncommon to encounter individuals who remain robust and active well into their later years, and you too can achieve this through dedication to fitness.

Regular exercise doesn't just help you retain muscle; it also keeps your metabolism at a healthy rate, providing you with the strength and endurance needed to tackle daily tasks. While the support of loved ones becomes increasingly important as you age, staying fit reduces your reliance on others, allowing you to maintain your independence.

Moreover, regular physical activity plays a crucial role in preventing unexpected falls, a significant concern for older adults. By staying active and maintaining strong muscles, you can reduce the risk of falls and the associated injuries, promoting a healthier and more confident lifestyle.

Incorporating regular exercise into your life isn't just about aesthetics; it's about preserving your vitality and well-being as you journey through the different stages of life.

Enhancing Digestive Health

Regular exercise contributes significantly to your overall well-being, including your digestive health. Incorporating a consistent workout routine into your lifestyle benefits your digestive tract by strengthening it and promoting gut health.

Physical activity helps maintain the healthy flow of your intestinal processes, preventing sluggishness. The advantages of exercise for digestion are both immediate and long-term.

Exercise can also provide relief from common digestive discomforts such as gas, heartburn, constipation, and stomach cramps. However, it's essential to note that excessive or ill-timed physical activity can have adverse effects on digestion, leading to issues like abdominal pain, constipation, heartburn, bloating, and an upset stomach.

To maximize the digestive benefits of exercise, consider working out before a meal rather than immediately after eating. Timing plays a critical role in ensuring your body's equilibrium during physical exertion.

The reason exercising immediately after a meal can hinder digestion is the redirection of blood flow to aid in the digestion process within the stomach and intestines. When you engage in physical activity too soon after eating, blood is diverted away from the digestive organs back to your muscles, potentially causing digestive discomfort. Therefore, it's advisable to schedule your workouts thoughtfully to complement your digestive well-being.

Enhancing Your Physical Appearance

Regular exercise can work wonders for your appearance, and it accomplishes this in various ways. Two significant factors that contribute to a more youthful and attractive appearance are muscle development and skin improvement.

Exercise plays a pivotal role in enhancing the condition of your skin by promoting detoxification. When you engage in physical activity, you stimulate your body's natural sweating process. Sweating efficiently allows your skin to expel toxins through your pores, acting as a natural detoxification method. This means that with regular exercise, you may find less need for external detoxifying treatments or medications.

According to Audrey Kunin, a dermatologist based in Kansas City, engaging in regular exercise is akin to giving yourself a mini-facial. She explains that vigorous exercise causes your pores to dilate, effectively expelling sweat and oil that may be trapped within them.

However, it's crucial to follow your exercise routine with proper skincare practices, including washing your face immediately after your workout. Failure to do so could result in the reabsorption of sweat and oils into your pores, potentially causing skin issues.

Moreover, consistent exercise contributes to stress reduction, which in turn can have a profound impact on your appearance. Both mental and physical exhaustion can accelerate the aging process, making you appear older than you are.

By establishing and maintaining a regular workout plan, you can give yourself a more youthful and vibrant outlook.

Additionally, muscle development resulting from exercise can provide a substantial boost to your appearance. As you build muscle, your clothing fits better, enhancing your overall silhouette and boosting your self-confidence when you step out.

Incorporating exercise into your daily routine not only benefits your internal health but also leaves a positive mark on your external appearance, offering you a healthier and more youthful glow.

Enhancing Mental Performance and Boosting Work Productivity

Success in today's fast-paced, technology-driven world often requires a calm and focused mind, particularly when tackling mentally demanding tasks. In this modern era, where computer-based work is prevalent, maintaining your concentration is paramount.

Yet, distractions often abound, making it challenging to excel. Fortunately, regular exercise offers you the essential tranquility to not only survive but thrive in your daily endeavors.

Unlocking Greater Efficiency

Enhanced relaxation leads to improved efficiency. It's essential to understand that subpar performance won't propel you to the pinnacle of your career or help you realize your full potential.

In today's hyper-competitive environment, there's immense pressure to deliver exceptional results or risk losing your position to the myriad of individuals waiting to seize opportunities and outperform. Whether you're an employee or an entrepreneur, staying relevant and excelling is non-negotiable.

The relentless competition that characterizes the business world demands that you remain sharp at all times. Engaging in stress-relieving activities, such as regular workouts, provides you with a significant advantage. It clears the mental clutter, allowing you to approach your tasks with a sharp and unclouded mind.

The Power of Clarity

Imagine having the mental clarity to dissect complex problems, formulate innovative solutions, and execute tasks with precision. This is the power that regular exercise can bestow upon you. It grants you the clarity needed to navigate the challenges of a high-stakes, fast-paced world.

In essence, engaging in a consistent workout routine serves as the foundation for mental resilience. It empowers you to tackle even the most demanding tasks with composure and efficiency, ensuring that you stay ahead in an environment that values top performance. By investing in your physical well-being, you're investing in your mental prowess, and ultimately, your success.

CHAPTER 4: UNLOCKING THE SCIENTIFIC WONDERS OF PHYSICAL FITNESS

Dr. Cheng once remarked that if the myriad benefits of exercise could be encapsulated into a pharmaceutical, it would command a price tag of a million dollars. Scientists have long been intrigued by the transformative effects of regular physical activity, and their investigations have yielded promising insights. Let's delve into some of the remarkable discoveries in this realm.

Empowering the Immune System

In a groundbreaking study, researchers illuminated the profound impact of a mere 20-minute moderate workout on the immune system. This investigation engaged the participation of 47 healthy volunteers, each assigned to either jog or walk on a treadmill, tailored to their fitness levels. Before and after their exercise sessions, the scientists closely monitored levels of a key inflammatory marker known as TNF.

The results were nothing short of remarkable. Post-exercise, a discernible 5% reduction in the quantity of immune cells responsible for producing TNF was observed. This finding underscores the potency of exercise in modulating our immune responses, providing us with yet another compelling reason to embrace physical fitness.

This study's findings illuminate the potential of physical activity to fortify the immune system by curbing excessive inflammation. Researchers unequivocally established the anti-inflammatory properties of exercise.

However, the precise mechanisms governing this phenomenon remained elusive. It's essential to recognize that inflammation constitutes a natural immune system response to injuries and illnesses. Nonetheless, when inflammation spirals out of control, it can become counterproductive, ushering in discomfort and various adverse effects.

Consequently, the study's revelation that exercise possesses anti-inflammatory benefits bears considerable significance. It underscores the capacity of physical activity to shield against chronic conditions resulting from overactive inflammatory responses.

This discovery is truly empowering, suggesting that individuals may not necessarily need to rely on anti-inflammatory medications to mitigate the risk of excessive inflammation. In line with Dr. Cheng's assertion, the advantages of regular exercise appear to be invaluable, potentially worth far more than a million dollars.

Reducing Cancer Risk

Cancer, a devastating disease afflicting people worldwide, poses significant challenges in terms of treatment, often involving costly surgeries with various side effects. Consequently, prevention emerges as the most effective strategy. Encouragingly, one powerful method to reduce the risk of cancer is regular exercise.

Numerous studies have illuminated the connection between routine physical activity and a reduced incidence of breast and colon cancer. A comprehensive review of multiple studies has underscored that moderate physical activity offers a more significant protective effect compared to lower-intensity activities.

Remarkably, physically active individuals, both men and women, exhibit a substantial 30%–40% decrease in the risk of developing colon cancer, with women enjoying a notable 20%–30% reduction in breast cancer risk.

This systematic review compellingly confirms that engaging in regular exercise is strongly associated with a decreased prevalence of specific cancers, particularly breast and colon cancer. Additionally, the research reinforces the notion that cancer patients who participate in recreational physical activities are less likely to succumb to the disease compared to their less active counterparts.

Preventing Cardiovascular Disease

Regular exercise significantly benefits overall health by elevating your heart rate. Research indicates that women, in particular, enjoy a reduced risk of mortality from diseases associated with physical inactivity, notably cardiovascular disease. Studies have solidified the link between regular exercise and decreased mortality risk from heat-related illnesses in both men and women.

For example, a comprehensive eight-year study examined the impact of exercise on middle-aged individuals' health. The results revealed that individuals with the lowest levels of physical fitness faced an elevated risk of death from cardiovascular disease.

Conversely, those in the highest fitness quintiles experienced a notable reduction in mortality risk. Recent investigations have further illuminated this relationship, indicating that being physically fit or active results in over a 50% reduction in the risk of death from heart-related illnesses.

Crucially, these studies have unveiled the stark contrast faced by physically inactive middle-aged women who engage in less than one hour of exercise per week. They face a staggering 52% increase in all-cause mortality and a concerning 29% spike in cancer-related mortality compared to their physically active counterparts.

These findings emphasize the pivotal role of exercise in preventing cardiovascular diseases and promoting overall well-being.

Decreasing the Risk of Diabetes

Diabetes can have a profound negative impact on your life, from personal discomfort to dietary restrictions. However, the good news is that regular exercise can be a powerful shield against this debilitating disease. Scientific research has unveiled the significant role that workouts play in diabetes prevention.

For example, a study involving 46 participants engaged in energy-expending activities found that both aerobic and resistance exercises effectively reduce the risk of developing type 2 diabetes.

The researchers made a striking discovery: regular exercise can decrease the risk of type 2 diabetes by as much as 6%. This benefit was particularly evident among participants with a high body mass index (BMI), who are at a higher risk of diabetes.

This study not only emphasized the importance of weight loss but also demonstrated that exercise itself significantly reduces the likelihood of becoming a diabetes patient. Multiple studies have reinforced these findings, lending credence to the reliability of these results.

In another study involving 271 male physicians, similar outcomes were recorded. Participants who engaged in weekly physical activities that induced perspiration experienced a reduced incidence of type 2 diabetes.

Remarkably, these active individuals also exhibited a lower risk of cardiovascular ailments, highlighting the wide-ranging benefits of regular exercise in safeguarding overall health.

Enhancing Bone Health

If you're looking to bolster your bone density, incorporating regular exercise into your routine is crucial. Weight-bearing exercises, especially resistance training, have a profound impact on bone mineral density.

A comprehensive review of numerous cross-sectional reports unequivocally demonstrated that engaging in resistance training leads to increased bone mineral density. Consequently, individuals who partake in these activities are more likely to enjoy robust bone health.

Furthermore, the choice of sports or exercises you engage in plays a pivotal role in determining your bone mineral density. Athletes involved in high-impact sports tend to exhibit superior bone mineral density compared to those participating in low-impact activities.

Therefore, while exercise is beneficial for bone health across the board, specific routines yield more pronounced benefits. Similar findings have been corroborated by other researchers in studies involving individuals of various age groups, from children and adolescents to middle-aged and older adults.

Numerous longitudinal studies have explored the relationship between exercise and bone health across diverse populations. Although researchers advocate for further studies involving larger participant pools, the existing body of research strongly supports the assertion that physical activity not only improves bone health but also diminishes the risk of bone-related diseases.

Weight-bearing and impact exercises, in particular, are recognized as effective means of combating age-related bone loss, providing yet another compelling reason to incorporate exercise into your lifestyle.

CHAPTER 5: PHYSICAL FITNESS AND RELATIONSHIPS

Regular exercise offers a multitude of benefits, as highlighted in the previous chapter through science-based evidence. With these compelling reasons in mind, you already have a strong incentive to initiate and maintain a workout routine. However, it's worth noting that physical fitness also plays a significant role in enhancing your sex life.

Before delving into the connection between physical fitness and your sex life, it's essential to emphasize that exercise should not be pursued solely to improve sexual prowess and adventures. While these benefits exist, it's important to view exercise as a holistic practice that contributes to overall health and well-being. This chapter explores how staying fit can positively impact your intimate relationships.

Attracting the Opposite Sex

Attraction is a multifaceted concept, and what individuals find attractive can vary widely. Some are drawn to intelligence, while others are captivated by emotional intelligence. However, it's an undeniable truth that physical appearance often plays a pivotal role in sparking initial interest. Human nature tends to assess individuals based on their outward appearance, creating a first impression that influences subsequent interactions.

While people must recognize and appreciate the qualities beyond physical appearance, it's equally important to acknowledge that a strong initial impression can open doors to deeper connections. Striving to enhance your physical appearance is not about vanity but about increasing your chances of being noticed for the wonderful qualities you possess beyond the surface.

Self-confidence is a vital aspect of attraction. By looking in the mirror and genuinely appreciating your physique, you boost your self-esteem and project confidence. Imagine being the best version of yourself, both inside and out, and consider how this transformation can impact your ability to attract potential romantic partners.

A Balanced Approach to Fitness

It's essential to reiterate that while improving your physical appearance is an admirable goal, it should not be the sole focus of your fitness journey. Exercise offers a wide range of health benefits, from improving cardiovascular health to enhancing mental well-being. These benefits should be at the forefront of your motivation to engage in regular physical activity.

In summary, physical fitness can indeed have a positive influence on your attractiveness and confidence, which, in turn, can enhance your romantic prospects. However, it's crucial to maintain a balanced perspective, realizing that the primary goal of exercise is to promote overall health and well-being.

By embracing this holistic approach, you'll not only improve your chances of attracting potential partners but also experience the numerous other benefits that come with a fit and healthy lifestyle.

Enhancing Self-Confidence in Dating

Confidence is an invaluable quality that can lead to success in various aspects of life, including your romantic endeavors. Low self-esteem can inadvertently lead to missed opportunities, as individuals with higher confidence levels tend to stand out and get noticed. In contrast, those with low self-confidence may find themselves overlooked, even by less qualified individuals.

When it comes to dating and relationships, self-confidence is your ally. It's the key to securing a date and navigating the intricacies of the dating scene effectively. A lack of self-confidence can lead to avoidable blunders that can sabotage potential connections.

For instance, recall the character Aladdin from the movie "Aladdin," who fumbled his chance to impress the princess due to his anxiety-induced words. This highlights the critical role self-assuredness plays in romantic pursuits.

Moreover, your physical appearance significantly contributes to your self-confidence, especially when interacting with the opposite sex. Striving for a physique that exudes attractiveness can boost your self-assurance, both in and out of the bedroom. When you possess a physique that you're proud of, it naturally translates into increased self-assurance in your intimate moments.

Maintaining Fitness and Libido

Physical activity has a profound impact on sexual function, either positively or negatively, depending on your approach. Research from the University of California has shown that regular exercise can significantly enhance sexual performance and lead to more satisfying orgasms for both men and women. This correlation also extends to women, who experience similar benefits from physical activity.

Another study from the University of Texas explored the connection between physical fitness and sexual performance.

Their findings indicated that exercise increases physiological sexual arousal in women. Essentially, women who engage in regular physical activity are more likely to experience heightened arousal compared to those who don't exercise. This is attributed to the increased heart rate, improved breathing, and heightened muscular activity that result from physical exertion.

However, it's essential to strike a balance. Excessive exercise can have a detrimental impact on your sex life. Research conducted by scientists from the University of North Carolina at Chapel Hill revealed that men who engage in strenuous, high-intensity exercise routines may experience decreased libido. This suggests that men who opt for lower-intensity workouts might enjoy better sexual performance compared to their counterparts who overexert themselves.

In summary, enhancing self-confidence in dating is crucial for building meaningful connections, and maintaining fitness can positively influence sexual performance. It's essential to strike the right balance in your exercise routine to reap the benefits without compromising your libido.

Enhancing Your Sex Life Through Exercise

When stress takes hold of your life, it can manifest in various ways, affecting both your physical and emotional well-being. Surprisingly, stress can also impact your sexual health and desires. This chapter explores the intricate relationship between fatigue, mental exhaustion, and your sex life, shedding light on how exercise can be the key to rejuvenating your libido.

The Stress Connection

When stress becomes a constant companion, it can sabotage your workout routine and dampen your libido. This is due, in part, to the hormone cortisol, which surges in response to stress and can diminish your interest in sex over time.

However, exercise offers a powerful antidote. Engaging in physical activity triggers the release of endorphins, commonly known as the "feel-good" hormones, which act to lower cortisol levels.

Reducing cortisol levels through exercise is a game-changer for your stress levels, ultimately boosting your sexual arousal and desire. Renowned expert Dr. Penhollow affirms that physical activity can significantly reduce depression, and it's no secret that sexual desires often wane when one isn't in a positive emotional state. By combatting depression, regular exercise can enhance your sex life by rekindling your desire.

Enhancing Sexual Performance through Exercise

Beyond improving your mood and reducing stress, exercise provides additional benefits that contribute to a satisfying sex life. Here are some ways in which exercise can enhance your sexual performance:

1. Improved Flexibility: Regular workouts enhance your flexibility, increasing your ability to explore and enjoy various sexual positions, leading to greater satisfaction.

2. Enhanced Strength: Some sexual maneuvers require physical strength and endurance. Engaging in regular exercise builds the physical vitality and power needed to engage in optimum sexual activity, ensuring you can fully enjoy intimate moments.

Exercises for a Boosted Sex Life

Certain exercises are particularly effective in boosting sexual performance and desire. Here are a few key activities to consider incorporating into your fitness routine:

Kegels

Kegel exercises strengthen pelvic floor muscles, which experts believe can enhance libido in both men and women. These exercises also address issues like bowel control and urine leakage. In women, strong pelvic muscles can lead to more powerful orgasms and even help delay ejaculation in men.

Strength Training

Strength training, which involves using weights or resistance, can significantly reduce stress levels and boost your overall mood. It provides a powerful counterbalance to the effects of stress on your sex life.

Walking

Simply taking a thirty-minute walk around your surroundings can have a profound impact on your sexual health. In men, it lowers the risk of erectile dysfunction by a remarkable 41%, as revealed by a Harvard study.

Swimming

Though not an everyday activity like walking, just thirty minutes of swimming three times a week can work wonders for your sex drive, according to the same study. Additionally, swimming can lead to weight loss, which further contributes to your sexual well-being.

Incorporating these exercises into your routine can not only boost your physical fitness but also reignite the spark in your sex life, fostering a healthier and more satisfying intimate experience.

CHAPTER 6: CRAFTING AN EFFECTIVE WORKOUT PLAN

Working out at home offers numerous advantages, including saving money on gym transportation and providing the time for a proper warm-up before diving into your session. This chapter will guide you through the process of creating a feasible and effective home workout plan.

Starting with a Solid Foundation: Setting Clear Goals

To ensure a successful home workout journey, it's essential to set well-defined goals that will serve as your guiding light. Begin by asking yourself critical questions such as:

- Am I aiming to lose weight?
- Do I want to bulk up and build muscle?

Regardless of your fitness aspirations, it's crucial to commence with the simplest exercises. These initial exercises will not only help you build confidence but also prevent the risk of injuries from starting with overly strenuous routines. It's beneficial to document your fitness targets as they will later serve as both inspiration and motivation.

Designing Your Typical Home Workout Plan

Your workout plan should align closely with your fitness objectives. You may need to conduct additional research to identify exercises that best support your goals. As a beginner, a reasonable starting point is to work out three days a week. For instance, if you choose to exercise on Mondays, Wednesdays, and Fridays, a typical week's routine could look like this:

Workout 1: Monday

After a few minutes of warming up, you can begin your routine with the following activities:

Activity #1: Power Snatch

This exercise involves bending your knees while holding a dumbbell in one hand between your legs. Next, explosively extend your hips, knees, and ankles to raise the weight overhead. Drop into a half squat position to hold the weight overhead once your body is straight from head to toe, then stand up straight. It's recommended to rest for a minute before proceeding to the next activity.

By structuring your home workout plan with clear goals and a focus on gradual progression, you set yourself up for success while minimizing the risk of injuries. In the following chapters, we will delve deeper into various exercises and routines that align with specific fitness objectives, providing you with the knowledge and tools you need to achieve your fitness goals at home.

Activity #2: Squat Press

Start with dumbbells at shoulder level, ensuring a firm grip. Begin by descending into a squat position, maintaining proper form and balance. As you rise from the squat, use the power from your legs and core to press the weights directly overhead.

Exhale as you lift the dumbbells. Slowly lower the weights back to shoulder level, and return to the initial squat position. This compound exercise engages multiple muscle groups, promoting strength and coordination.

Activity #3: Jump Squat

After a brief sixty-second rest, position the dumbbells by your sides. Initiate the movement by descending into a half squat, ensuring your knees are aligned with your toes. Explosively jump upward from the ground, extending your body fully.

Softly land back in the squat position, absorbing the impact through your legs. Repeat the jump squat for a dynamic lower-body workout that enhances power and agility.

Activity #4: Windmill

Begin by holding a single dumbbell overhead with a strong and steady arm. Maintaining focus on the weight above, hinge at the waist and bend sideways, lowering the dumbbell along your leg. This exercise provides an effective core and oblique workout while improving flexibility and balance.

Activity #5: Roll-Out

Starting with dumbbells positioned just below your shoulders, kneel on the floor. Roll the weights forward as far as your core strength allows, maintaining control throughout the movement. Engage your abdominal muscles to control the return to the initial position. Both the roll-out and windmill exercises are exceptional for developing a sculpted and resilient core.

Workout 2: Wednesday

Similar to the first day, this workout emphasizes functional movements that are both effective and approachable. These exercises help maintain your momentum, even as fatigue sets in. The routine includes:

Activity #1: Dumbbell Swing

Hinge at the hips while holding the dumbbell with a firm grip. Swing the dumbbell between your legs and use your powerful hip drive to raise it to shoulder height. Maintain a controlled motion throughout. Reverse the movement to return to the starting position, and smoothly transition into the next repetition.

The dumbbell swing is an excellent full-body exercise that enhances strength and cardiovascular endurance. Rest for one minute between exercises to optimize performance and recovery.

Activity #2: Overhead Squat

This exercise focuses on maintaining proper form while performing a challenging movement. Begin by holding a dumbbell in each hand directly overhead, arms fully extended. Next, initiate the squat by bending at your hips and knees simultaneously, keeping your back straight and chest up. It's crucial to ensure that you don't allow the weights to drift forward during the descent. This exercise emphasizes balance, mobility, and control.

Activity #3: Press-Up Renegade Row

Engage your upper body and core with this compound exercise. Start with a dumbbell in each hand, and assume a push-up position with your wrists aligned under your shoulders. As you perform a push-up, maintain stability by holding the dumbbells.

After completing the push-up, row one dumbbell up to your side while keeping your body in a straight line. Alternate by rowing the other dumbbell up while lowering it back to the floor, completing one repetition.

Activity #4: Side Lunge

Enhance your lower body strength and flexibility with the side lunge exercise. Begin by gripping a dumbbell in each hand. Take a big step to the side, bending your leading knee while keeping your foot pointing forward and your knee aligned with your toes.

Push off your leading foot to return to the starting position and then repeat the movement in the opposite direction. Alternate sides with each repetition to work both legs evenly.

Activity #5: Leg Raise

Strengthen your core and lower abdominal muscles with the leg raise exercise. Lie on your back, holding a dumbbell securely between your feet, with your heels slightly elevated off the ground. With your legs straight, raise them vertically while maintaining control. Slowly lower your legs without allowing your heels to touch the floor. This exercise provides an excellent challenge for your core muscles.

Workout 3: Friday

In this final workout of the week, it's recommended to tackle more technically demanding exercises to end on a high note. These exercises may not necessarily be the heaviest or most complex but require exceptional mobility and control.

Activity #1: Back of Steel

Initiate this exercise by lowering into an overhead squat with dumbbells held above your head. Gradually lower the weights to shoulder level while remaining in a squat position. Continue by repeating the lowering and pressing movement while maintaining your squat position, emphasizing control and stability.

Activity #2: One-Leg Squat

Hold dumbbells by your sides and stand on one leg to perform this challenging single-leg squat. Bend at the hips and knees while keeping your chest upright, then press back up to the starting position. Complete all repetitions on one leg before switching to the other, focusing on balance and control.

Activity #3: Woodchop Lunge

Begin by placing a dumbbell over one shoulder. As you lunge forward with the opposite leg, simultaneously bring the weight diagonally down across your body. Swap sides after completing all repetitions on one side, engaging your core and legs throughout the movement.

Activity #4: One-Leg Romanian Deadlift

Stand on one leg with dumbbells hanging by your thighs. Lower the weights toward the floor by hinging at your hips while keeping them close to your leg. Avoid leaning too far forward to prevent strain on your lower back. Maintain balance and control as you perform this exercise.

Activity #5: Turkish Get-Up

End your workout session with the highly beneficial Turkish Get-Up. Begin by lying on the floor, holding a weight above your face. Progressively raise by bending your knee on that side and coming up onto your elbow, then your hand, and pushing your hips off the floor.

Bring your straight leg back under your body and remove your hand from the floor as you stand up. This exercise demands both strength and coordination, making it a rewarding challenge.

This Friday workout routine is designed to push your boundaries and enhance your overall fitness level.

CHAPTER 7: CREATING AN EFFECTIVE DIET PLAN

An effective workout plan goes hand-in-hand with an excellent diet plan. Exercise is a physical activity that requires energy, and your diet plays a crucial role in providing that energy. Furthermore, your eating habits directly impact your overall appearance and well-being. This chapter is dedicated to guiding you in creating a diet plan that complements your workout routine.

The Connection Between Physical Fitness and Dietary Habits

Physical activity is like the engine of a car, and your body requires fuel to run efficiently. Therefore, the importance of a well-balanced diet in your workout plan cannot be overstated. As you engage in exercise, you'll become fitter and potentially lose weight. However, your energy requirements will also change. As an active individual, you'll need an adequate amount of the following nutrients:

- Carbohydrates: The body's primary source of energy.
- Fat: An additional source of vitality.
- Protein: Vital for the maintenance and repair of tissues, including muscles.
- Water: Critical for replacing fluids lost during physical activities.

To ensure you have these essential nutrients, you should maintain a moderate, varied, and balanced diet. Moderation means consuming a bit of everything without excess. You can incorporate all essential food groups into your diet without overindulging in any one category. Variety involves consuming different types of foods to ensure you receive a wide range of nutrients. No single food provides all the necessary nutrients, so diversify your choices to avoid overconsumption of any specific substance. Balance entails eating the recommended servings from each food group most days.

It's important to note that athletes and highly active individuals have unique nutritional requirements due to the demands they place on their bodies. They often require more carbohydrates, such as grains, compared to the average person. However, their protein needs may not be as high as others.

Carbohydrates are stored in the liver and muscles as readily available energy, and this energy is quickly depleted during exercise. Endurance athletes, such as cyclists and runners, require a substantial amount of carbohydrates because of the nature of their activities. They should consume carbohydrates before or during exercise since the body has limited storage capacity for this nutrient.

A Sample Diet Plan

This book includes a two-week diet plan scientifically designed for significant weight loss, offering approximately 1250 calories daily, which is suitable for physically active individuals. Below is a summary of the fundamental dietary guidelines:

Vegetables: One and a half cups (options include starchy veggies, orange veggies, dry beans, dark green veggies, and peas).

Oils: Four teaspoons (choices include vegetable oil, light salad dressing, butter, or low-fat mayo).

Fruit: One cup (options include various fruits like pears, apples, mangoes, cherries, grapes, raspberries, strawberries, blueberries, and pomegranates).

Grains: Four ounces (equivalent to bread, cereal flakes, muffins, cooked rice, or dry pasta).

Milk: Two cups (yogurt, milk, soy milk, or cheese).

Meats and Beans: Three ounces (lean poultry, meat, fish, eggs, peanut butter, cooked beans, nuts, or seeds).

Remember to mix and match food items throughout the day while staying within your caloric goal. You can also follow one of the pre-designed menus provided to ensure you're on the right track.

Nutritional Guidelines

Vegetables: Consume one and a half cups daily, including options like starchy veggies, orange veggies, dry beans, dark green veggies, and peas.

Oils: Limit oils to four teaspoons daily, choosing from vegetable oil, light salad dressing, butter, or low-fat mayo.

Fruit: Enjoy one cup of fruit daily, with choices ranging from pears, apples, mangoes, cherries, grapes, raspberries, strawberries, blueberries, and pomegranates.

Grains: Consume four ounces of grains daily, including options like bread, cereal flakes, muffins, cooked rice, or dry pasta.

Milk: Aim for two cups of dairy or dairy alternatives daily, such as yogurt, milk, soy milk, or cheese, preferably low-fat or non-fat options.

Meats and Beans: Include three ounces of lean protein sources daily, such as poultry, meat, fish, eggs, peanut butter, cooked beans, nuts, or seeds.

This well-structured diet plan, coupled with your workout routine, will help you achieve your fitness goals efficiently and sustainably.

↓ Menu #1: Energizing Day

Breakfast (8 am – 9 am)

One slice of whole-grain toast

Refreshing Berry Smoothie (Blend one cup of soymilk, ice cubes, and one cup of assorted berries)

A touch of butter (one teaspoon)

Lunch (11 am – 1 pm)

A colorful assortment of steamed vegetables (about three-quarters cup, including carrots, broccoli, cauliflower, etc.)

Nutrient-packed grain (one cup, choose from brown rice, white rice, wild rice, millet, quinoa, etc.)

Lean protein (two ounces, approximately the size of half a deck of playing cards)

Snack (3 pm – 4 pm)

Choose between a half ounce of seeds or a protein-rich egg

Dinner (5 pm – 7 pm)

Two teaspoons of a light, flavorful dressing

A generous portion of leafy greens (about one and a half cups)

Creamy delight: One and a half ounces of cheese

↓ Menu #2: Wholesome Choices

Breakfast (8 am – 9 am)

Creamy yogurt (one cup)

A hearty serving of oatmeal (half a cup)

Complement with herbal tea or a soothing black coffee

Lunch (11 am – 1 pm)

A slice of whole-wheat bread

A fresh medley of tomato, cucumber, and lettuce (equivalent to a three-quarter cup total)

Protein-packed tuna (two ounces)

Lightly dressed with a teaspoon of olive oil and a teaspoon of mayo

Snack (3 pm – 4 pm)

Satisfy your cravings with a juicy piece of fruit or a cup of fresh, vibrant fruit

Dinner (5 pm – 7 pm)

One corn tortilla

A crunch of shredded lettuce (half a cup)

Top it off with zesty salsa (half a cup)

Nourishing black beans (half a cup)

Melt-in-your-mouth cheese (half an ounce)

A side of comforting cooked rice (half a cup)

↓ Menu #3: Balanced Nourishment

Breakfast (8 am – 9 am)

A nourishing start with half a cup of milk or soy milk

Dive into a bowl of high-fiber cereal (one cup)

Sweeten it up with the natural goodness of a ripe banana

Lunch (11 am – 1 pm)

Crisp, raw veggie sticks (one cup of carrot sticks, celery, or green peppers)

Satisfying pasta (one cup)

Drizzle with two teaspoons of heart-healthy olive oil

Lean protein (two ounces) to keep you fueled

Snack (3 pm – 4 pm)

Choose between half a cup of fresh vegetables or half a cup of pasta sauce to curb your cravings

Dinner (5 pm – 7 pm)

A creamy delight: One cup of low-fat cottage cheese

Pair with six wholesome crackers

Indulge a bit with a half-ounce of mixed nuts for added crunch and flavor

These enhanced menus offer a balanced and delicious approach to your daily meals, ensuring you stay energized and satisfied throughout the day.

Tips for Dieting Success

Embarking on a strict diet plan can be challenging, but with the following carefully crafted strategies, you can increase your chances of achieving success:

1. Weekly Planning

Take time to plan your meals and snacks for the week ahead. Having a structured meal plan in place can help you stay on track and avoid impulsive food choices.

2. Eliminate Temptations

Clear your fridge and pantry of any foods that might tempt you to stray from your diet plan. Removing these temptations makes it easier to stick to your dietary goals.

3. Stay Hydrated

Aim to drink at least eight glasses of water daily. Having a glass of water before each meal can reduce your appetite and prevent overeating by giving your brain time to signal fullness.

4. Mindful Eating

Practice mindful eating by savoring each bite and eating slowly. Put your fork or spoon down between bites to help you recognize when you're satisfied. Remember, it takes approximately 20 minutes for your brain to register fullness.

5. Explore New Foods

Introduce variety into your diet by trying new foods and recipes. This can make your restricted diet more interesting and enjoyable.

6. Spice It Up

Enhance the flavor of your meals with spices and herbs. This not only adds excitement to your dishes but can also increase your satisfaction and reduce the urge to overeat.

7. Home Cooking

Cooking your meals at home allows you to have greater control over ingredients and portion sizes. This makes it easier to adhere to your diet plan and resist the temptation to overindulge outside.

8. Post-Meal Ritual

After finishing a meal, brush your teeth to deter snacking and signal the end of eating for the time being. This simple practice can help prevent unnecessary calorie intake.

9. Prioritize Sleep

Lack of sleep can trigger increased appetite and overeating. Prioritize getting adequate sleep to support your weight loss goals and overall well-being.

10. Keep Your Objective in Mind

Above all, never lose sight of your ultimate objective. Remind yourself regularly why you embarked on this dietary journey, and use it as motivation to stay committed to your goals.

By incorporating these practical tips into your dieting plan, you can increase your chances of success and achieve the results you desire while maintaining a healthy relationship with food.

CHAPTER 8: MAINTAINING YOUR PLAN AND MOMENTUM

Starting something new is relatively easy, but the real challenge lies in sticking to a plan and achieving your goals over time. You may have devised a diet and workout plan after reading this book, but as days turn into weeks, you might encounter reasons to quit.

There will be moments when discouragement creeps in, and the thought of continuing may seem daunting. However, you can ensure that you stay on track and maintain your consistency by employing the following strategies.

Consistency in Time and Location

When you act once, it's just an act. But when you perform it regularly, it becomes a habit. The human mind and body are remarkably adaptable, and you can train yourself to develop a craving for certain activities. Just like brushing your teeth or taking a daily shower, you can condition your body to perceive your home workout plan in a similar light.

The key to achieving this is consistency in both time and location. Try to maintain the same time of day and the same workout spot whenever possible. When you consistently perform an activity at a specific time and place, your body adapts to it.

You'll find yourself eagerly looking forward to that time, almost as if something is missing on days when you skip it. While alarms may help initially, after a week or two of consistent workouts, your body will naturally remind you that it's time. Even if you forget temporarily, you'll likely recall it later in the day because it has become an integral part of your daily routine.

Reminding Yourself of the Benefits

There's little point in doing something if you don't do it consistently and effectively. Consistency is especially critical in the realm of workouts. You can't achieve your desired physique if you're inconsistent in your exercise routine. Whether your goal is weight loss or muscle building, staying consistent is essential.

To maintain focus and motivation, it's crucial to constantly remind yourself of the benefits of your fitness journey. Begin by writing down your goals from the outset, making them easily accessible for regular reflection. Consider setting them as reminders on your phone or placing them as short notes in visible spots around your home to serve as constant reminders. Your environment can be a powerful tool for setting yourself up for success.

For instance, if you use a workout mat, place it near your bed before you sleep to serve as a visual cue for the next morning's exercise. These are just a few examples, but creativity in finding ways to remind yourself is key. Motivation alone may wane on certain days, but by consistently reminding yourself of your goals, you can inspire and commit yourself to staying on track.

In conclusion, achieving and maintaining your fitness goals requires both initial motivation and ongoing commitment. Remember that motivation may ebb and flow, but by reminding yourself of what you aim to achieve and by establishing consistent routines, you can stay committed and inch closer to your desired results.

Maintain a Progress Journal

Cultivating the habit of keeping a journal offers a multitude of benefits. Among these advantages is the ability to keep your thoughts organized, providing a platform to record your daily musings, emotions, and significant events.

If you aspire to refine your writing skills, journaling can serve as an invaluable tool. It encourages you to articulate specific topics, develop your ideas, and thereby enhance your writing prowess. However, journaling goes beyond improving your writing; it can significantly aid in achieving your fitness goals.

Your journal serves as an ideal repository for your goals, including your workout objectives. Each time you update it, you revisit your goals, rekindling your determination and commitment to follow through on your fitness plan.

Furthermore, it offers a convenient and practical means to track your progress. Documenting your milestones fosters excitement and motivation to keep moving forward. You can readily identify your next target and strategize how to attain it.

Moreover, maintaining a journal allows you to capture ideas on the fly. You can jot down novel tips that may enhance your adherence to your diet and workout regimen. Location and time constraints become inconsequential when you have a journal at your disposal. Additionally, the act of updating your journal can be therapeutic, providing a channel to vent anxieties and frustrations, rather than carrying them within your mind. This practice contributes to your overall well-being by relieving stress and tension.

Share Your Achievements with Like-Minded Individuals

Discussing your pursuits with others not only reflects your dedication but also solidifies your commitment. The more you engage in conversations about your objectives and experiences, the more resolute you become in your pursuit. Therefore, it is crucial to share your fitness plans, progress, and achievements with individuals who share your interests and can provide valuable support.

However, exercise caution when selecting individuals with whom you share your workout journey. Past interactions can reveal those who may not align with your goals or values. Sharing your aspirations with individuals who do not appreciate the value of exercise might lead to discouragement.

As mentioned previously, if finding like-minded individuals in your immediate vicinity proves challenging, consider joining online communities or social media groups dedicated to fitness. These platforms offer a wealth of individuals who range from beginners to advanced fitness enthusiasts. You can glean insights from their experiences, learn from their challenges, and continuously improve your exercise routine.

Engaging with these platforms also offers you a valuable chance to connect with others, and share your journey, including both successes and challenges. Here, you'll effortlessly discover a treasure trove of tips and insights to enhance your progress.

Moreover, you'll come to understand that you're not alone in facing similar obstacles. Should you have any inquiries or uncertainties, these platforms become a wellspring of knowledge, providing you with the guidance you need to refine your fitness plan. And when you achieve a significant milestone, these spaces provide a platform to spread your joy and accomplishments among individuals who share your fervor and dedication.

CONCLUSION

In your pursuit of any goal, the lack of quality information can be a significant hindrance. This book has provided you with the essential knowledge needed to create and maintain an effective home workout plan. However, knowledge alone is insufficient for success; it must be accompanied by unwavering commitment and action.

The information you've gained is the foundation upon which your fitness journey is built, but it becomes meaningful only when put into practice. It's not enough to simply gather tips for your regular exercise routine; you must follow through with dedicated effort.

As you've learned, setting clear goals is crucial, but the benefits of a home workout plan extend far beyond the achievement of those objectives. Improved sleep, stress relief, reduced depression, and a decreased risk of cancer and diabetes are just a few of the scientifically supported advantages.

Embarking on and persisting with your workout plan is a choice that aligns with your overall well-being and future success. It's a path toward realizing the body shape you desire, enhancing your self-confidence, and excelling in various facets of your life.

Furthermore, maintaining your fitness can lead to improved sexual performance, contributing to greater satisfaction in your intimate relationships. By doing so, you can sidestep unnecessary attention and the hurtful ridicule that sometimes accompanies weight-related issues.

Remember, determination knows no bounds. You have the power to transform yourself and embrace a new lease on life. The decision to commence your workout and diet plan today is a declaration of your commitment to personal growth and overall wellness. Embrace this journey, and you'll discover a more vibrant, confident, and resilient version of yourself waiting on the horizon.